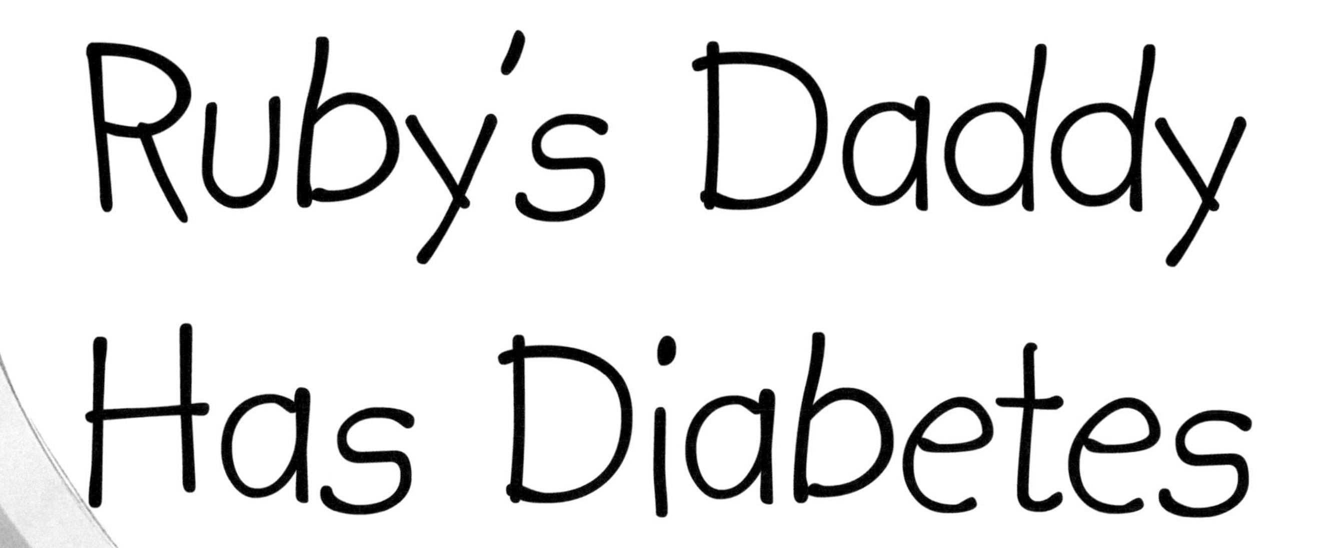

Ruby's Daddy Has Diabetes

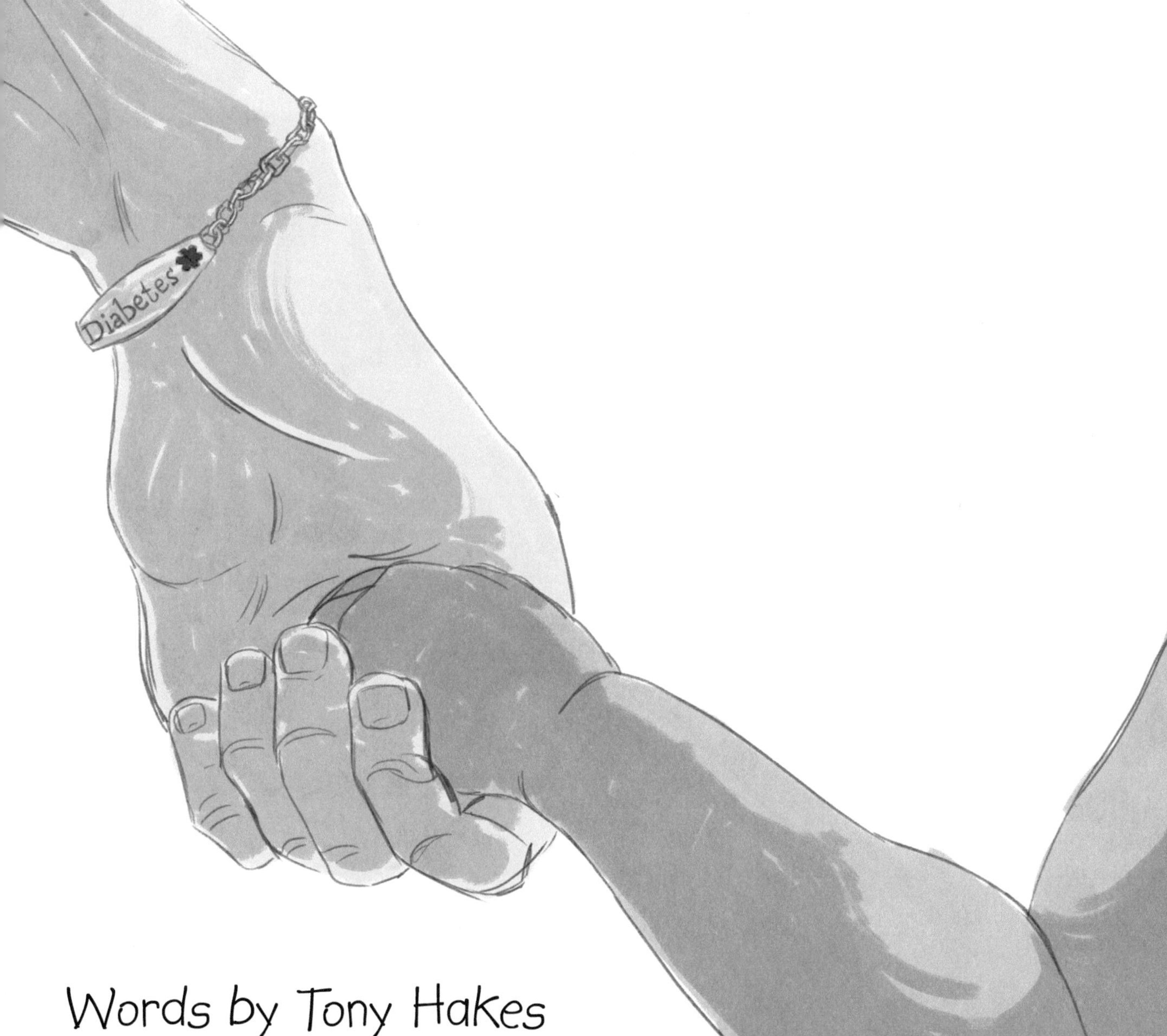

Words by Tony Hakes
Pictures by Monica Schubick

RUBY'S DADDY HAS DIABETES

iUniverse books may be ordered through booksellers or by contacting:

iUniverse
1663 Liberty Drive
Bloomington, IN 47403
www.iuniverse.com
844-349-9409

ISBN: 978-1-5320-7435-6 (sc)
ISBN: 978-1-5320-7436-3 (e)

Library of Congress Control Number: 2019942651

Print information available on the last page.

iUniverse rev. date: 11/17/2023

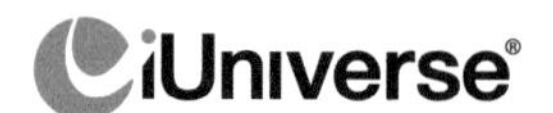

Ruby's Daddy Has Diabetes

Words by Tony Hakes
Pictures by Monica Schubick

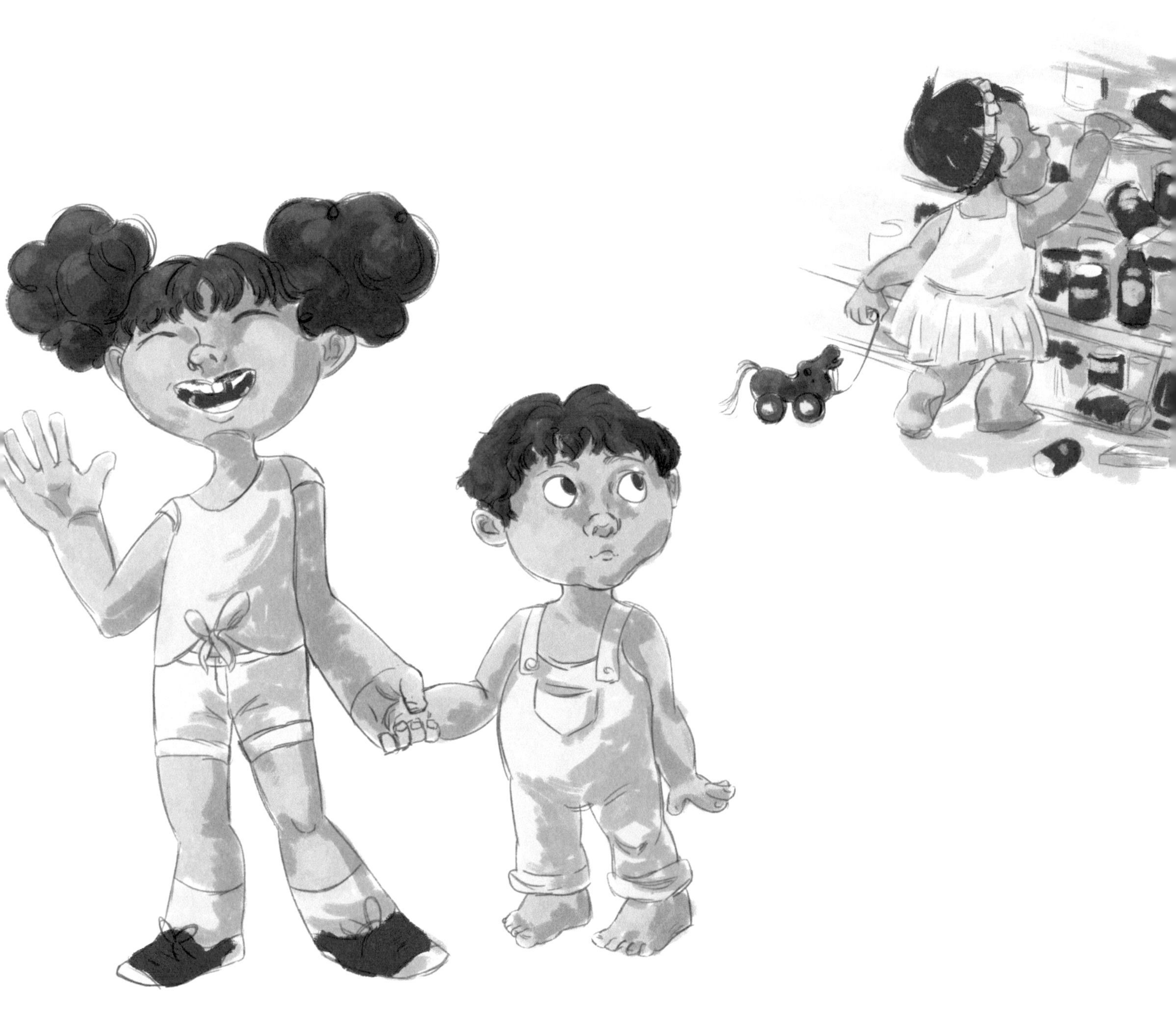

Hello, my name is Ruby, and I am five years old. I am in preschool and love going to ballet class. I also love playing at the beach and reading books. I'm very good at taking care of my younger brother Milo and my even-younger sister Lola.

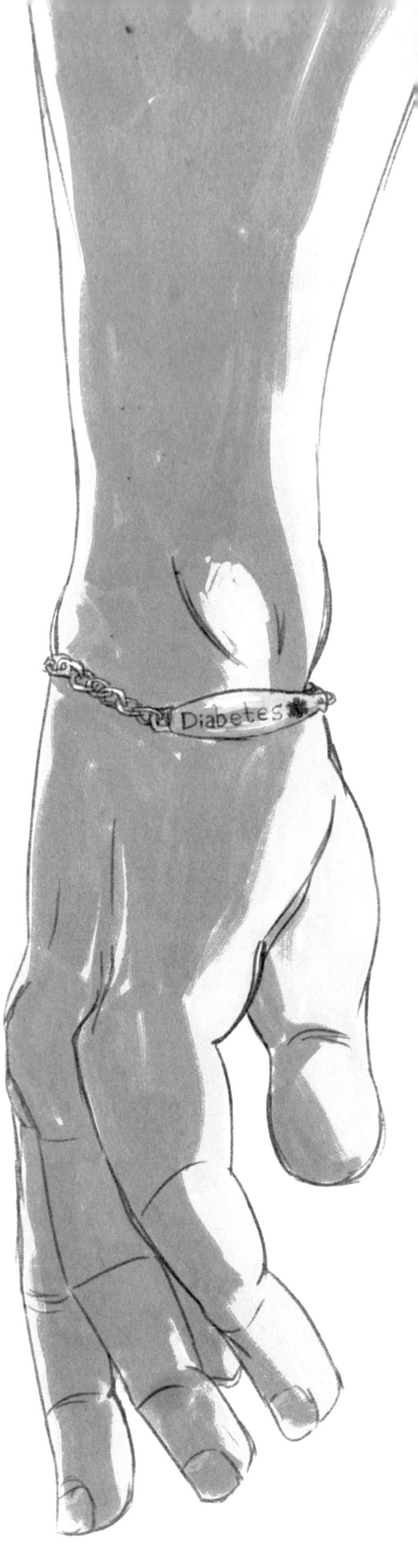

I have to help take care
of my daddy, too.

He has dia-bee-teez.

Dia-bee-teez means my daddy can't have very much sugar. Sugar is in lots of things like cake, ice cream, and brownies. I like sugar, but I try not to have too much of it. Sugar is not very good for you. Sometimes my daddy has too much sugar and he gets very tired and wants to take a nap, even if it's daytime!

That's why I make sure things he eats are sugar-free, which means they don't have any sugar in them. My younger brother Milo says he wants dia-bee-teez too, but Daddy says, "No, you don't!"

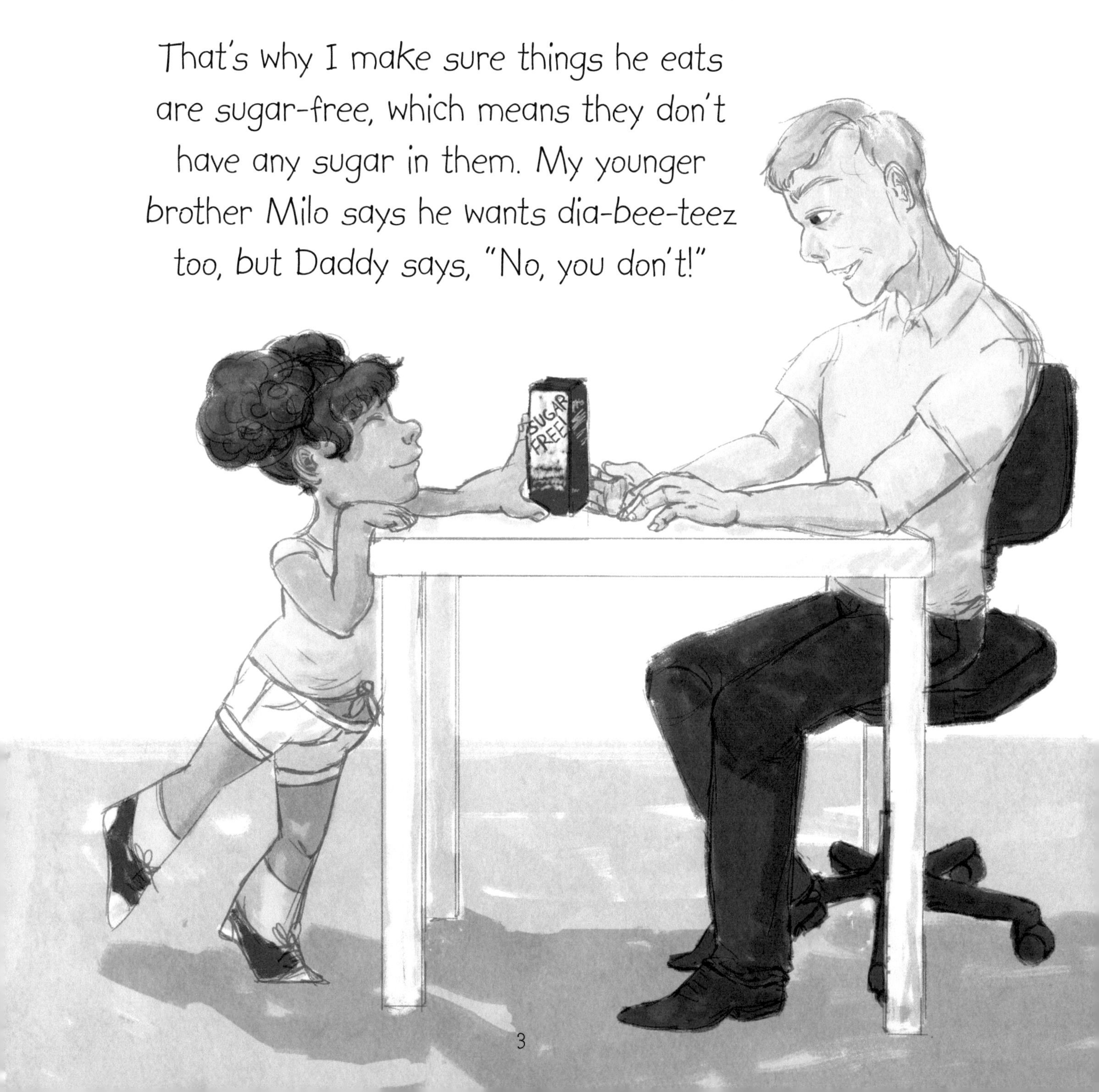

My daddy eats lots of fruits and vegetables. I am very "petite" for my age, but Daddy says I make up for it in personality. Whatever that means. He says eating fruits and vegetables will make me big and strong. I like fruits and vegetables, especially oranges and broccoli. Most of the kids in my preschool don't like broccoli, but I want to be big and strong too, so I eat lots of broccoli.

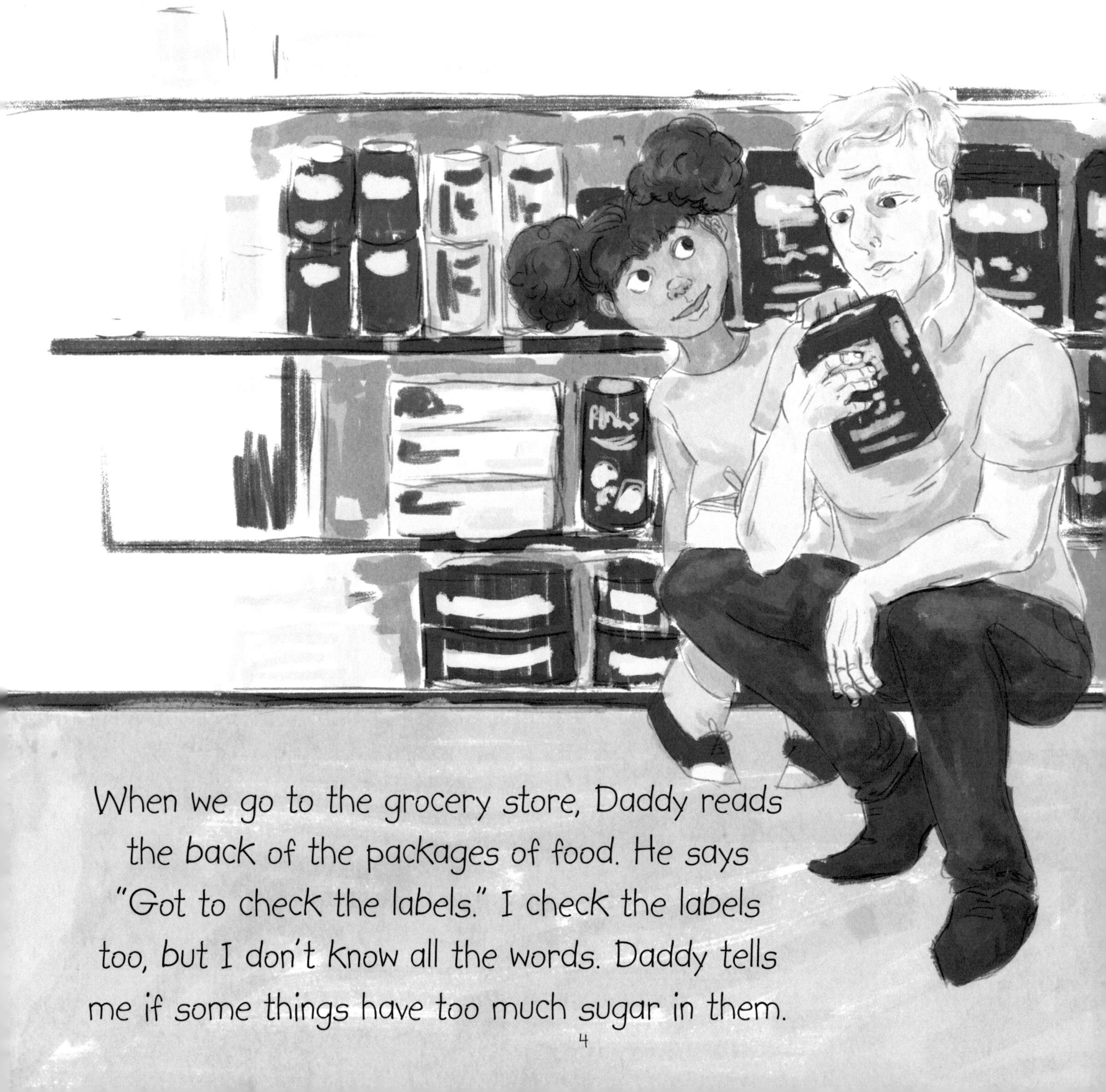

When we go to the grocery store, Daddy reads the back of the packages of food. He says "Got to check the labels." I check the labels too, but I don't know all the words. Daddy tells me if some things have too much sugar in them.

When my daddy goes to work, he works in an am-blee-ants. That's a special truck that takes people to the hospital when they are sick or hurt. He saves lives. I want to save lives when I get bigger too.

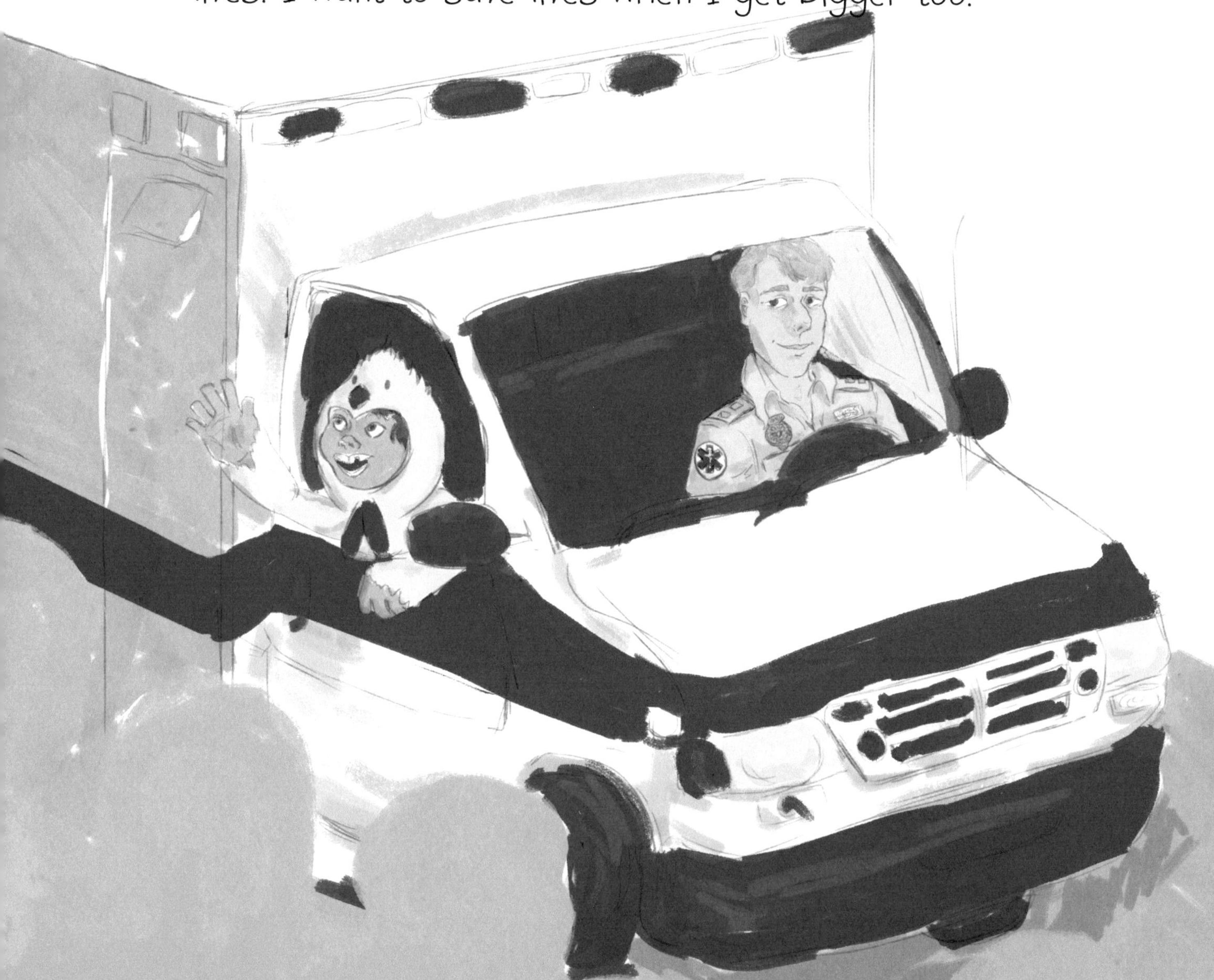

We had to call an am-blee-ants when my even-younger little sister fell. Mommy said Daddy might even need an am-blee-ants someday. Daddy says I already help him and my younger brother and even younger sister. Daddy calls me his "little guardian angel" because I help take care of everyone. Sometimes he lets me ride in the am-blee-ants. I got to ride in the am-blee-ants for a parade once. It was for Halloween and I wore my chicken costume.

Because of his dia-bee-teez, my daddy has to take special medicine called insulin. He takes the insulin by giving himself a shot in the stomach five times every day. I push the button to give him the medicine sometimes. I don't like shots. When I was little, I got four shots at the doctor's office. I tried not to cry, but the last one hurt really bad, and I cried a little. Daddy never cries when he gets a shot.

He also has to poke his finger five times every day. He bleeds a little bit, and puts the blood in a machine that tells him if he's had too much sugar.

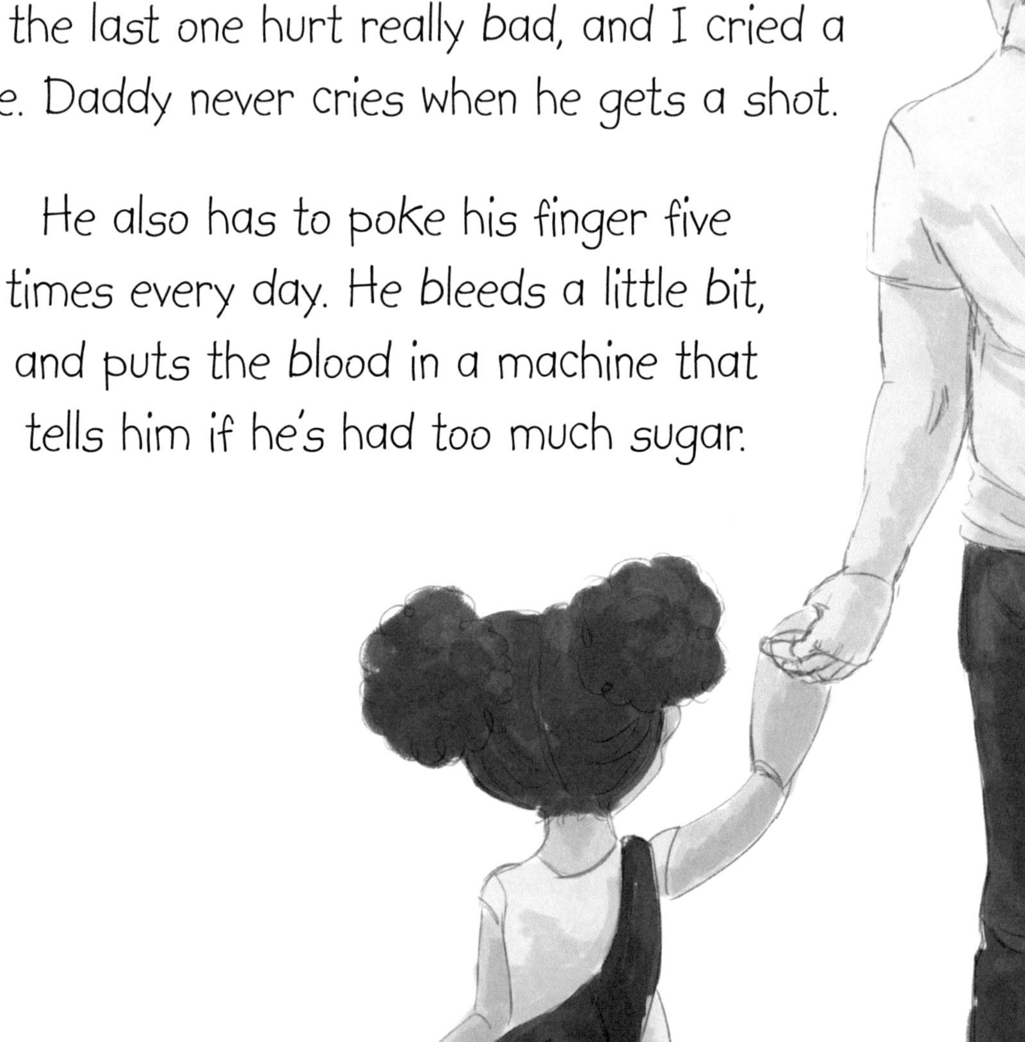

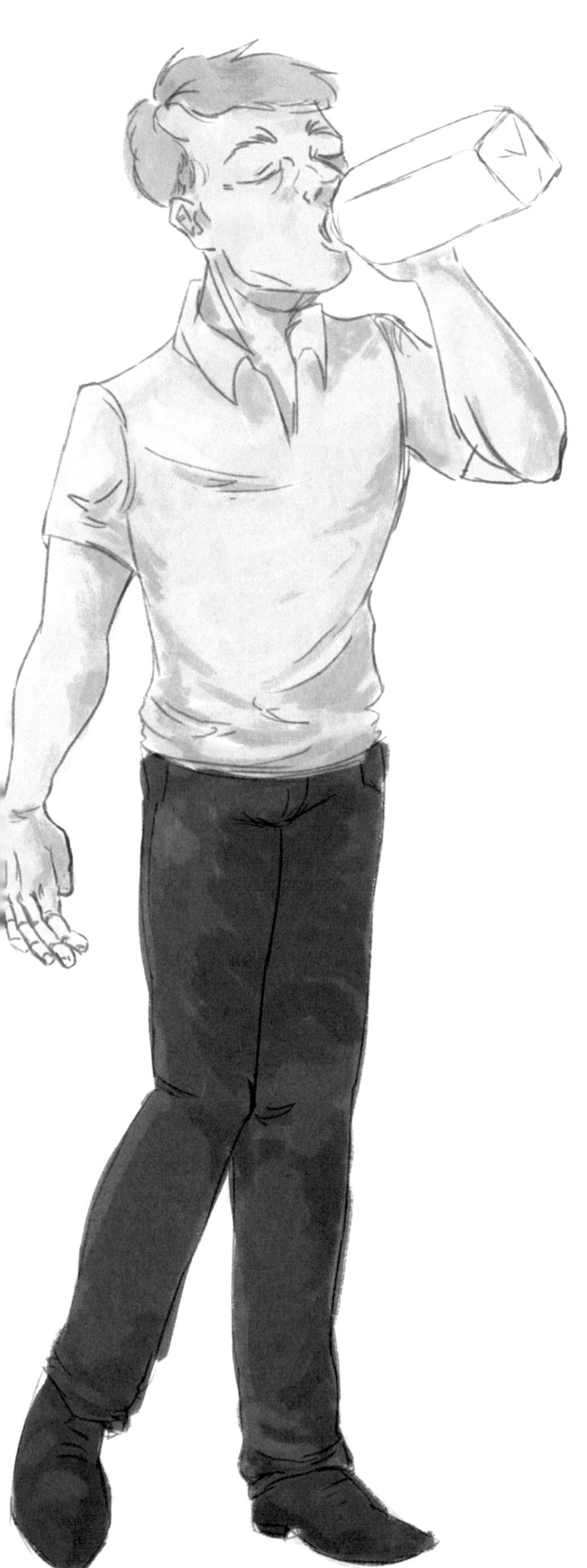

One time, Daddy had too much insulin and he was acting funny. He didn't know where he was, even though he was at our house. Mommy tried to talk to him, but he was very sweaty and shaking. He didn't even know his name! Mommy was worried, but she knew what to do. All Daddy needed was some milk.

Milk has lots of sugar in it, but Mommy says Daddy needs sugar when he has too much insulin. Mommy told me to do the same thing if Daddy ever acted that way again. Daddy keeps sugary snacks everywhere, just in case. Sometime I find them in his Jeep and in the laundry room. He even has some on his motorcycle! I like it when daddy shares his snacks with me.

Sometimes Daddy has a "low" and will drink right out of the carton! He says it's okay to drink out of the carton when you have dia-bee-teez. My little brother must have heard him 'cause he tries to drink out of the carton all the time. I've had to get milk for Daddy before, but the jug was so heavy that I dragged it on the floor for some of the way. I guess I have to eat more broccoli.

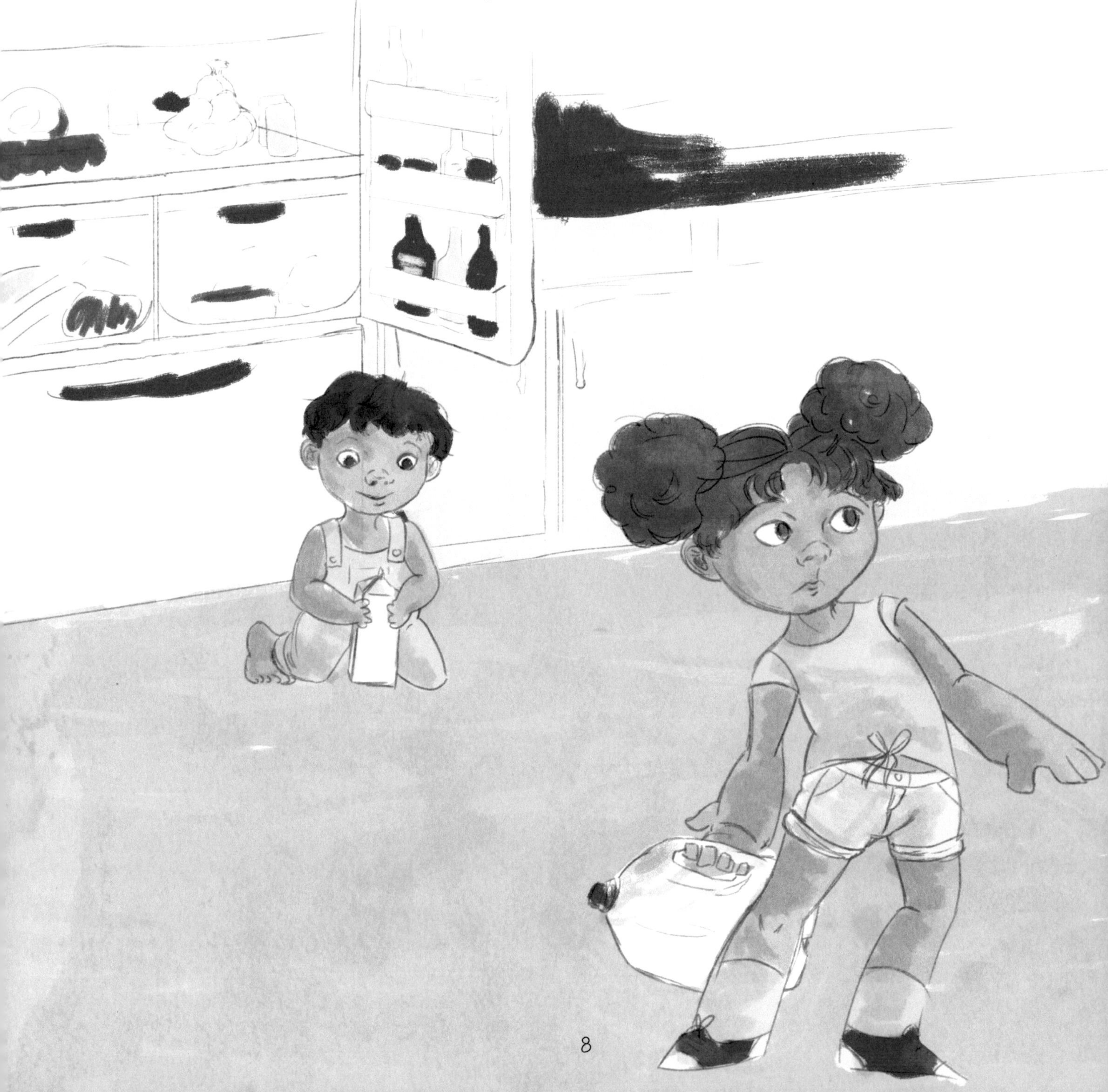

When we go out to eat I always get the macaroni and cheese. That's my favorite. When Daddy orders, he asks lots of questions, but the restaurant doesn't always have the right kind of food for Daddy and we have to go somewhere else. Mommy sneaks some food in for Daddy which makes me feel better. He likes to drink sodas that end with "zero". He lets me taste them, but they tickle my nose too much. My little brother Milo loves sodas that end in "zero".

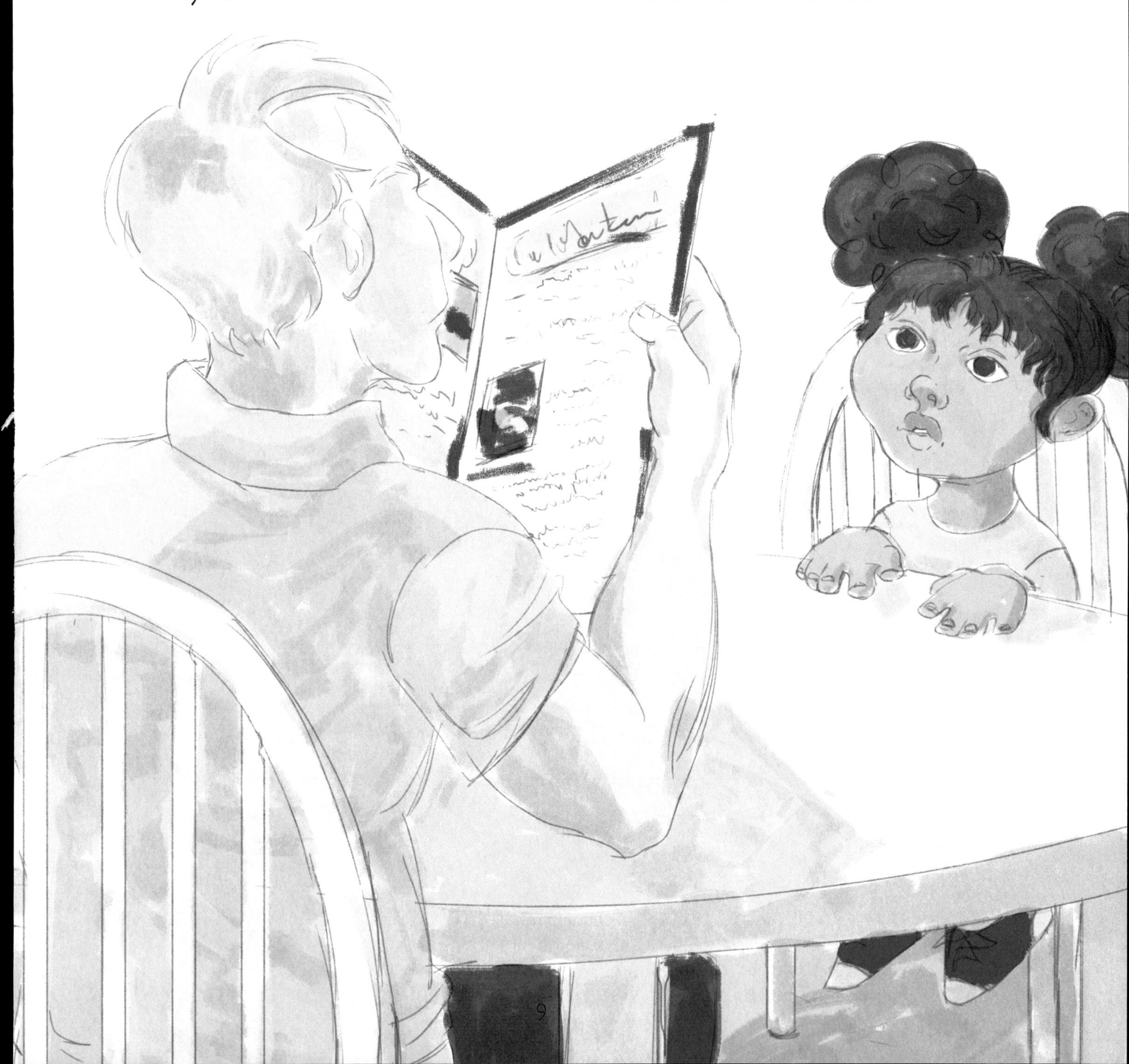

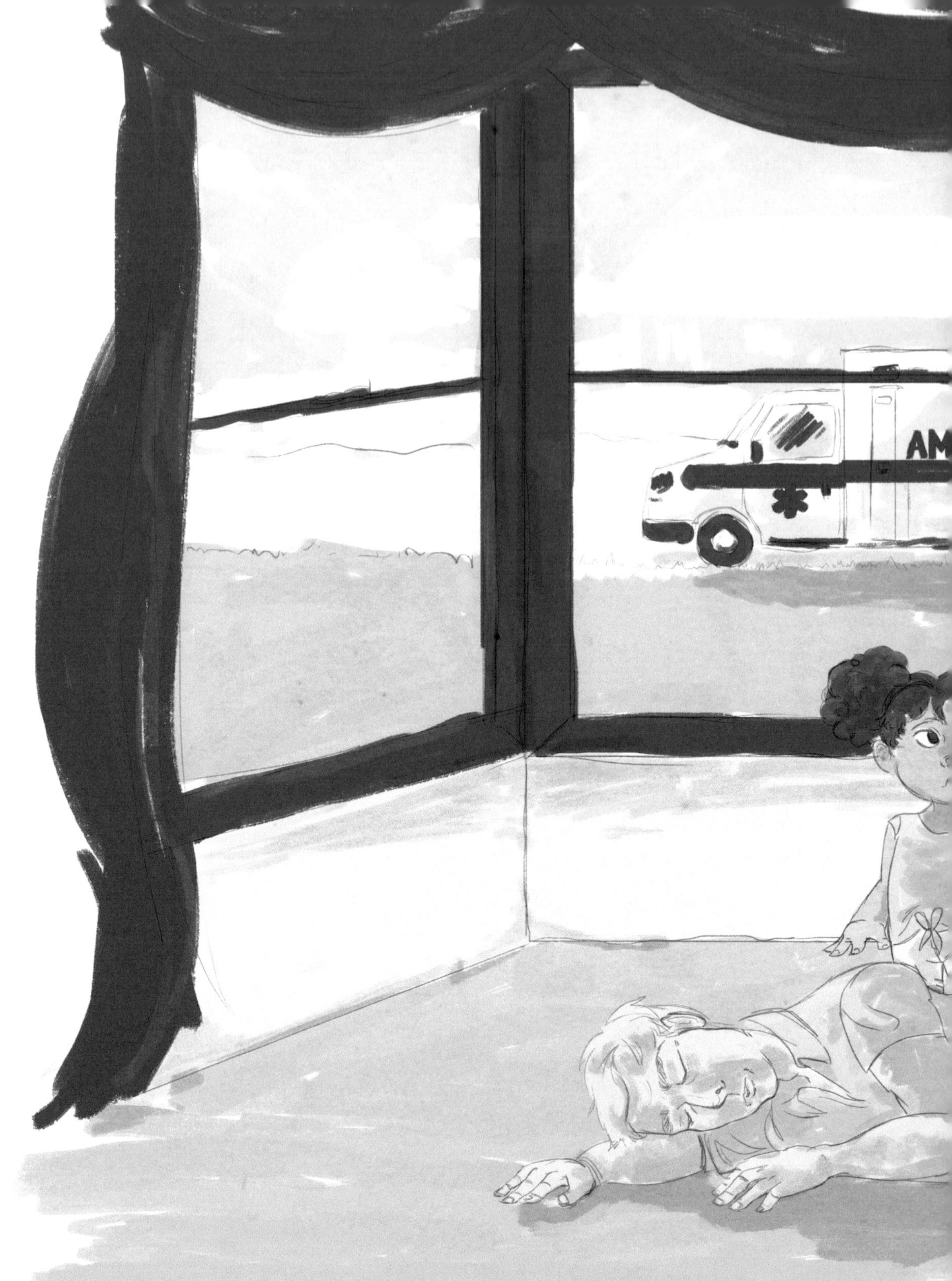

I found daddy on the floor once and he wouldn't wake up. Mommy wasn't home, but Daddy had taught me what to do. I used the phone to call a special number. I told them "My Daddy won't wake up, he has dia-bee-teez." They told me they would send an am-blee-ants to our house. I made sure my younger brother and even younger little sister were safe, then I waited by the door.

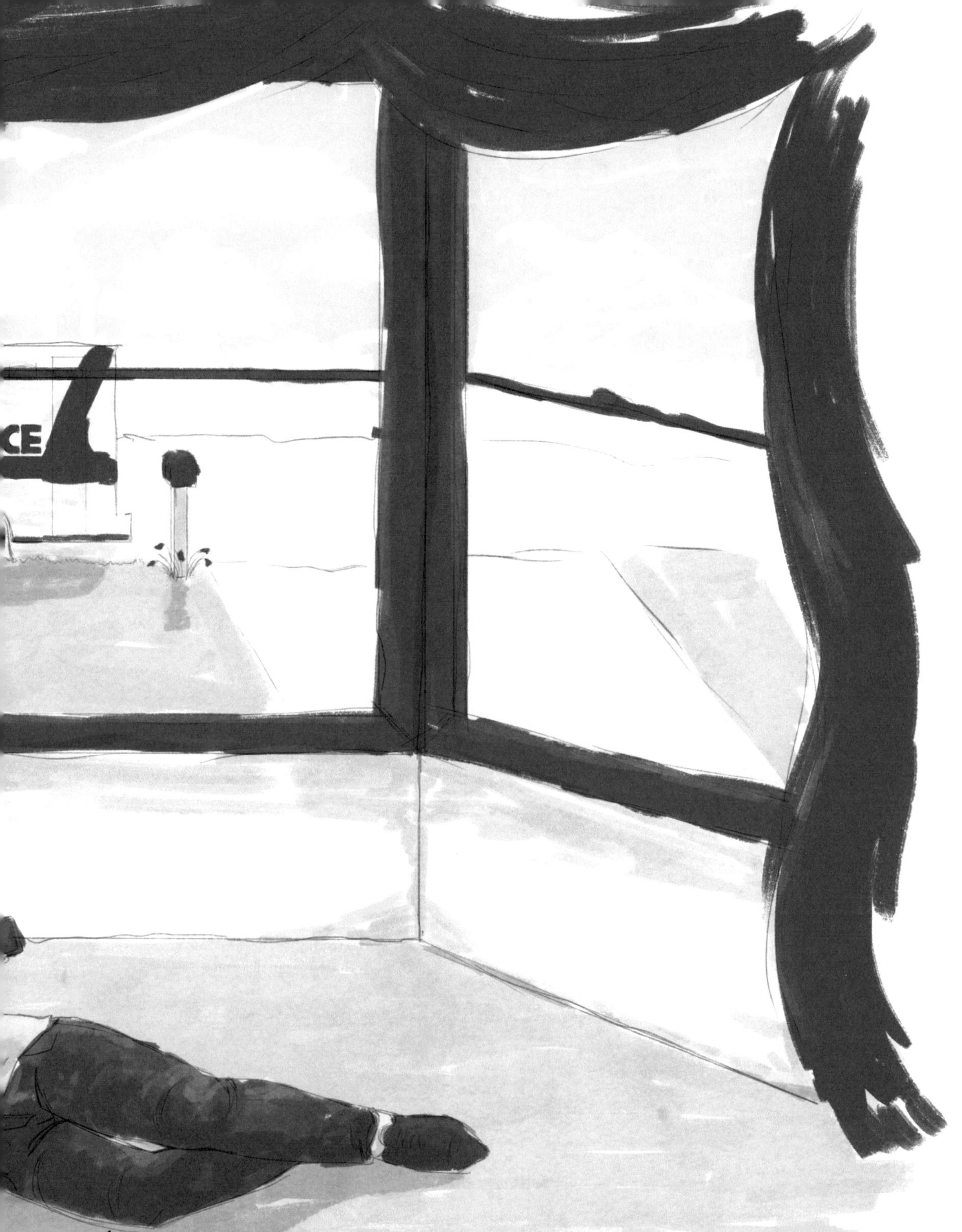

Police officers came first, which Daddy said would happen. I let them in and showed them where my daddy was. They used walkie-talkies to tell the am-blee-ants what was happening. When the am-blee-ants got there, they gave daddy special medicine, and he started to wake-up. A fire truck came too, which daddy said would also happen. The police officers called mommy and she came home right away.

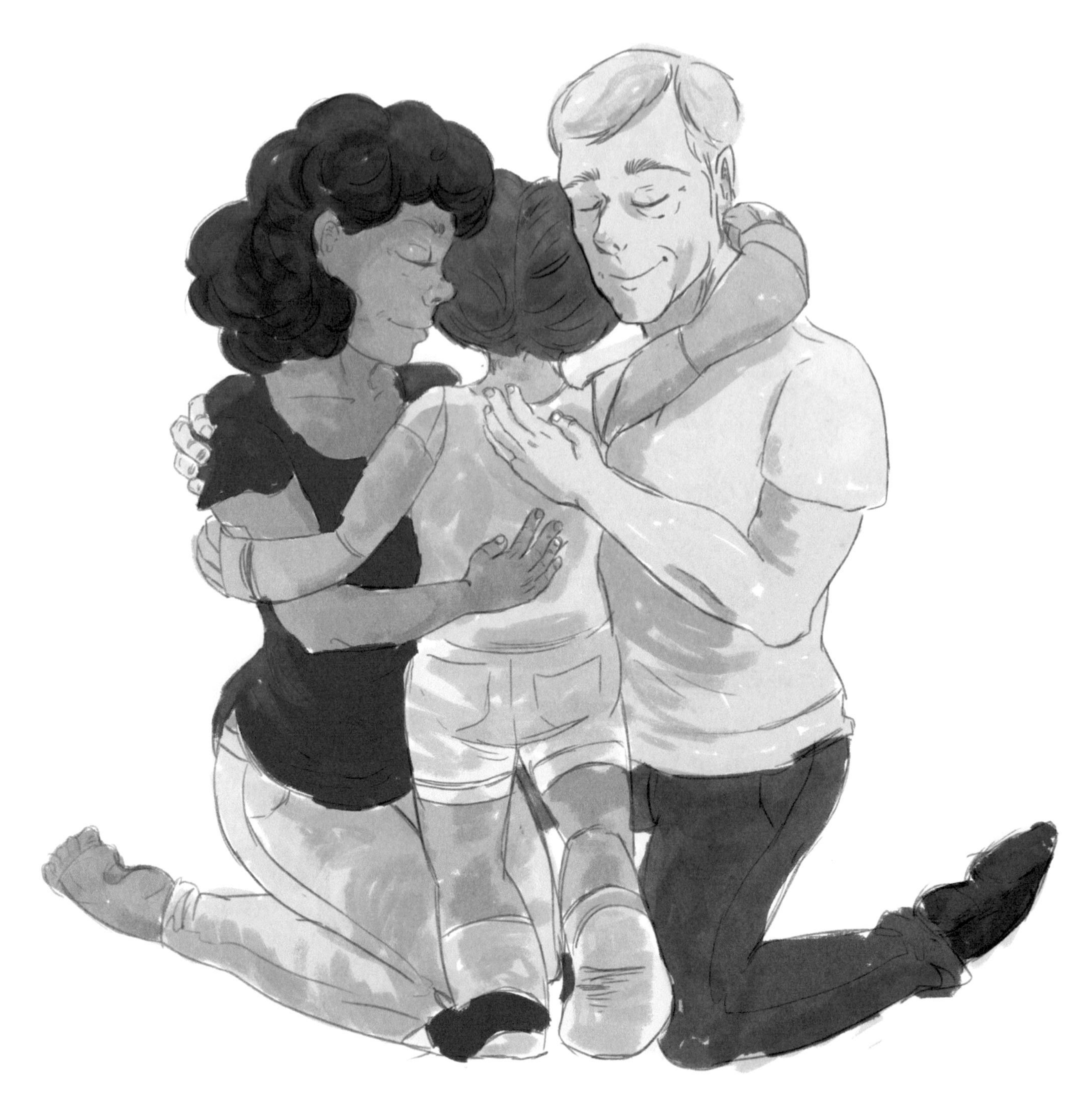

It was scary having all those people at our house, but Daddy said they were just trying to help him. Even though Daddy was okay, they still took him to the hospital to get "checked out". The policeman stayed with us until Mommy got home. She was really proud of me and gave us all hugs. Daddy came home later and wasn't sick anymore. He was really proud too and gave us all hugs too, even Mommy.

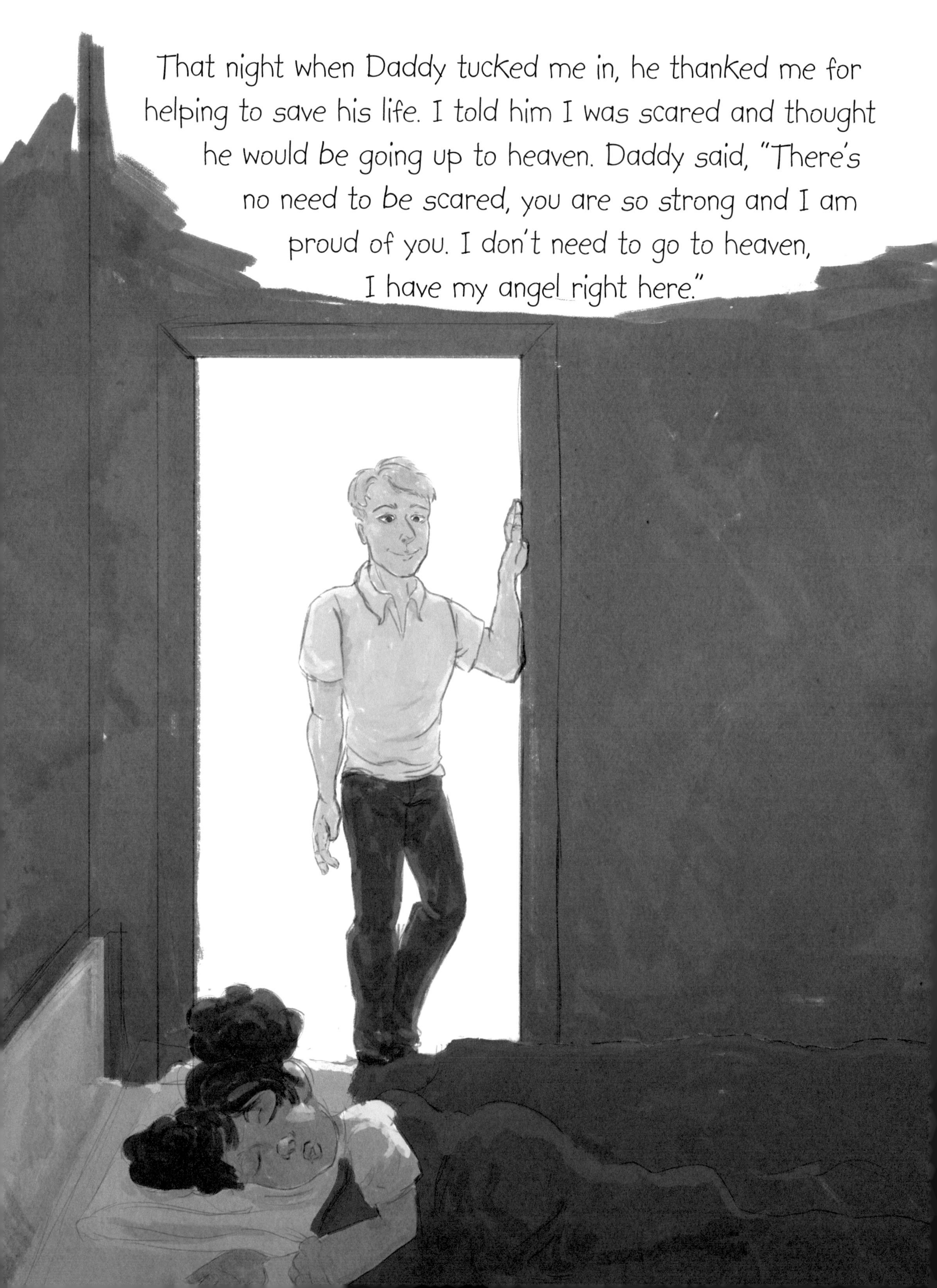
That night when Daddy tucked me in, he thanked me for helping to save his life. I told him I was scared and thought he would be going up to heaven. Daddy said, "There's no need to be scared, you are so strong and I am proud of you. I don't need to go to heaven, I have my angel right here."

About the Author

Tony Hakes lives in Iowa and enjoys spending time with his family, exploring the outdoors and motorcycling. This is his first book.

Notes

Notes

Notes

Notes

Printed in the United States
by Baker & Taylor Publisher Services